OXFORD MEDICAL PUBLICATIONS

Child Health: the Screening Tests

PRACTICAL GUIDES FOR GENERAL PRACTICE

Editorial Board

J. A. Muir Gray, Community Physician,
Oxfordshire Health Authority.
Ann McPherson, General Practitioner, Oxford.
Michael Bull, GP Tutor, Oxford.
John Tasker, GP Tutor, North Oxfordshire.

Forthcoming

Child Health
The Screening Tests

Practical Guides for General Practice 11

by

AIDAN MACFARLANE
Community Paediatrician,
Oxfordshire Health Authority

SUE SEFI
Research and Resource Officer,
Oxfordshire Health Authority

MARIO CORDEIRO
Paediatrician, Lisbon

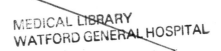
Oxford New York Tokyo
OXFORD UNIVERSITY PRESS

Oxford University Press, Walton Street, Oxford OX2 6DP
Oxford New York Toronto
Delhi Bombay Calcutta Madras Karachi
Petaling Jaya Singapore Hong Kong Tokyo
Nairobi Dar es Salaam Cape Town
Melbourne Auckland
and associated companies in
Berlin Ibadan

Oxford is a trade mark of Oxford University Press

Published in the United States
by Oxford University Press, New York

British Library Cataloguing in Publication Data
Macfarlane, Aidan
Child health: the screening tests.—(Practical
guides for general practice; 11)
1. Children. Health. Assessment
I. Title II. Sefi, Sue III. Cordeiro, Mario IIII. Series
613'.0432
ISBN 0–19–261768–0

Library of Congress Cataloging in Publication Data
Macfarlane, Aidan, 1939–
Child health: the screening tests/by Aidan Macfarlane,
Sue Sefi, Mario Cordeiro.
(Practical guides for general practice; 11)
(Oxford medical publications)
Includes indexes.
1. Children—Diseases—Diagnosis. 2. Children—Medical
examinations. 3. Medical screening. I. Sefi, Sue. II. Cordeiro,
Mario. III. Title. IV. Series. V. Series: Oxford medical publications.
[DNLM: 1. Child Health Services—Great Britain. 2. Mass
Screening—in infancy & childhood.   W1 PR141NK no. 11/WS 141
M143c]
RJ50.M33 1989 618.92'0075—dc20   89–16026
ISBN 0–19–261768–0 (pbk.)

Printed by Dotesios Printers Limited
Trowbridge, Wiltshire

Contents

1 Child health surveillance

For the first time ever in this country there is a proposal for a National Child Health Surveillance Programme to be carried out throughout England and Wales (and possibly Scotland), recommended by a working party made up of representatives from the Health Visitors' Association, the Royal College of Nursing, the Royal College of General Practitioners, the British Paediatric Association, and the General Medical Services Committee of the British Medical Association (Hall 1989).

This present booklet has been written for Health Visitors, General Practitioners, Clinical Medical Officers, and Community Paediatricians undertaking to carry out the screening tests contained in the National Child Health Surveillance Programme, and describes exactly how the tests are done.

It starts by describing how the screening programme fits in with the rest of the child health surveillance programme, and with health education and health promotion, precisely what 'screening' means, and what the screening schedule is. There is a short statement of why neurodevelopmental screening is not recommended at the present time. The text then describes, for each screening test: the incidence of the problem being looked for; the possible aetiologies and risk factors; precise details of how to carry out the screening test; the ages at which to carry it out; the indications for referral; and the follow-up after referral.

2 Screening tests in the context of child health surveillance

Screening tests are only one part of child health surveillance, and child health surveillance is only one part of the many programmes for trying to maintain children's health. The place of screening tests in the general scheme of things can be represented diagrammatically as shown in Fig. 2.1.

Screening tests are however an important part of the overall programme, because if the screening tests are not carried out absolutely correctly and the appropriate referrals are not made, then:

(1) too many parents will be worried unnecessarily by too many children being referred as being in a high-risk category when they are not (false positives); and

(2) some parents will be falsely reassured by a badly performed screening test when their child really does have a problem, and the child should have been referred as being in the high-risk category (false negatives).

A further important aspect of screening tests is that they can be validated. At the present time much of what is carried out in the way of child health surveillance is difficult to assess in terms of whether it helps the health of children or not. Screening tests can and should be assessed on an on-going basis both at district and, even more, at local level. This entails:

(1) reviewing, by observation, how the tests are actually carried out in child-health clinics; and

(2) collecting information concerning: the number and age of children being identified in terms of each of the various problems that are being screened for; by whom

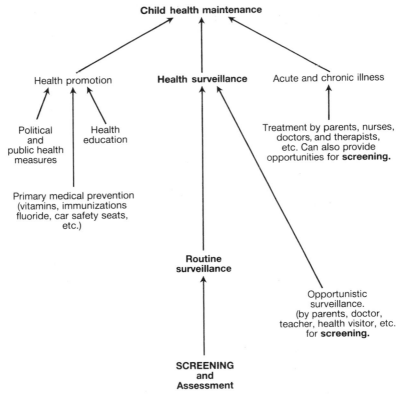

Fig. 2.1. The role of screening in an overall child health mainten-ance programme.

and by what means the problem was actually identified; and what the final outcome was after treatment.

The recent recommendations from the Joint Working Party on Child Health Surveillance (Hall 1989) are an important first step in developing an evaluative approach to the child-health service being provided, working towards the goal of every child's not only reaching his or her optimum level of health, but also maintaining that optimum.

3 Justifications for screening tests

Screening is the presumptive identification of unrecognized disease or defect by the application of tests, examinations, and other procedures which can be rapidly applied. Screening tests do NOT attempt to make a diagnosis. What they do is to separate out a group of individuals who are at 'high risk' of having the problem being looked for, from a group of individuals at 'low risk' of having the same problem. The principles on which to decide whether a test is a validated 'screening' test or not, were first defined by Wilson and Jungner (1968). These are:

(1) The condition being looked for should be an important health problem for the individual and for the community.
(2) There should be an acceptable form of treatment for patients with recognizable disease, or some form of useful intervention.
(3) The natural history of the condition should be known.
(4) There should be a recognizable latent or asymptomatic stage.
(5) There should be a suitable test or examination for detecting the disease in the latent stage.
(6) Facilities should be available for making the final diagnosis.

These conditions were then further elaborated by Cochrane and Holland (1969), who stated that screening tests should be:

(1) simple, quick, and easy both to perform and to interpret;
(2) acceptable to the person on whom the test is being performed;

(3) accurate;

(4) repeatable (high inter- and intra-observer reliability);

(5) highly specific (low false positives); and

(6) highly sensitive (low false negatives).

Only those tests that met these criteria were accepted by the Working Party—and they are the ones included in this booklet.

Neurodevelopmental assessments

Neurodevelopmental screenings using such standardized formats as the Denver Development Test, Griffiths, etc., have not been included because they do not meet the above criteria.

However, the neurodevelopmental status of a child should be assessed from parental observations and concerns, the child's medical history, and informal observations of the child's behaviour. Should this assessment give rise to concern then more formal testing should be carried out. References to some of the literature relative to neurodevelopmental testing are given at the end of this section.

Therefore, even though neurodevelopmental tests cannot be recommended for routine screening of all children on a regular basis, it still remains essential that those working in the field of child health surveillance should be able to carry out a neurodevelopmental test, should there be concern about a child's development.

Certain other tests which have in the past been used as 'screening tests' in certain parts of the country have also been reviewed, and subsequently excluded, on the grounds that they have not *yet* been validated by the criteria above.

These include attempts to screen the whole population for: scoliosis, hypertension, asthma, hypercholesterolaemia, haemoglobinopathies, psychiatric and behavioural disorders, proteinuria and bacteruria, cystic fibrosis, and Duchenne's muscular dystrophy.

In certain of these cases screening programmes have been extensively researched and found not to work; while others may well be validated in the future after further research has been done.

Who should carry out child health surveillance and screening?

Child health surveillance is carried out by a large number of people—parents, teachers, school nurses, relatives, health visitors, and doctors. It is both carried out on a routine (child-health clinic) and an opportunistic (surgery visits, in class, at home, etc.) basis.

The question as to who should carry out the 'screening' tests advocated *within* child health surveillance is answered by 'whoever has the appropriate training and skills'.

References

Cochrane, A. and Holland, W. (1969). Validation of screening procedures. *British Medical Bulletin*, **27**, 3–8.

Hall, D. (1989). *Health for all children. A programme for child health surveillance.* Oxford University Press.

Wilson, J. M. G. and Jungner, G. (1968). *Principles and practice of screening for disease*, Public Health Papers No. 34. WHO, Geneva.

Further reading on neurodevelopmental testing

Bellman, M. H., Rawson, N. S., Wadsworth, J., Ross, E. M., Cameron, S., and Miller, D. L. (1985). A developmental test based on the STYCAR sequences used in the National Childhood Encephalopathy study. *Child Care, Health and Development*, **11**, 309–23.

Borowitz, K. C. and Glascoe, F. P. (1986). Sensitivity of the Denver developmental screening test in speech and language screening. *Paediatrics*, **78**, 1075–8.

Cadman, D., Chambers, L. W., Walter, S. D., Feldman, W., Smith, K., and Ferguson, R. (1984). Usefulness of DDST to predict kindergarten problems in a general community population. *American Journal of Public Health*, **74**, 1093–7.

Camp, B. W. *et al.* (1977). Preschool developmental testing in prediction of school problems. *Clinical Pediatrics*, **16**, 257–63.

Egan, D. F. (1969). *Developmental screening 0–5 years.* Clinics in Developmental Medicine, No. 30. Spastics Society/Heinemann, London.

Eu, B. S. L. (1986). Evaluation of a developmental screening system for use by child health nurses. *Archives of Disease in Childhood*, **61**, 34–41.

Knobloch, H., Stevens, F., and Malone, A. F. (1980). *Manual of Development Diagnosis.* Harper and Row, Hagerstown.

Rutter, M. (1987). Assessment of language disorders. In *Language development and disorders* (ed. W. Yule and M. Rutter), pp. 295–311. Clinics in Developmental Medicine, Nos 101, 102. Mackeith Press/Blackwell, Oxford.

Silva, P. A. (1981). Predictive validity of a simple two-item screening test for three-year olds. *New Zealand Medical Journal*, **93**, 39–41.

Sonnander, K. (1987). Parental developmental assessment of 18-month-old children; reliability and predictive value. *Developmental Medicine and Child Neurology*, **29**, 351–62.

Sturner, R. A., Green, J. A., and Funk, S. G. (1985). Preschool Denver developmental screening test as a predictor of late school problems. *Pediatrics*, **107**, 615–21.

4 Summary of recommended screening procedures and assessments

Neonatal examination

- Review of family history, pregnancy and birth.
- Discuss any concerns expressed by the parents.
- Full physical examination, including weight and head circumference.
- Check for congenital dislocation of the hips.
- Check for testicular descent.
- Inspect eyes.
- Examine eyes for red reflex.
- If high risk of hearing defect—refer for further testing. Blood tests for phenylketonuria and hypothyroidism.

At discharge or within ten days of birth

- Check for congenital dislocation of the hips again.

Six to eight weeks

- Check history and ask about parental concerns.
- Physical examination, weight and head circumference.
- Check for congenital dislocation of the hips again.
- If status of testicular descent not known from birth information, or if not fully descended at birth—check again.
- Specifically enquire about parental concerns regarding hearing and vision.
- Inspect the eyes.

- Consider giving parents 'checklist' or 'questionnaire' for detection of hearing loss.

Seven to nine months

- Enquire about parental concerns regarding health and development.
- Ask specifically about vision and hearing.
- Check weight if indicated or parents wish it.
- Check for congenital dislocation of the hips.
- Check testicular descent if testes not previously recorded as being fully down.
- Observe visual behaviour and look for squint.
- Carry out distraction test for hearing.

Eighteen to twenty-four months

- Enquire about parental concerns, particularly regarding behaviour, vision, and hearing.
- Confirm that the child is walking with a normal gait.
- Confirm that the child is beginning to say words and is understanding when spoken to.
- *No* formal testing of vision and hearing but arrange detailed assessment if there is any doubt about either being normal.

Thirty-six to forty-two months

- Ask about vision, squint, hearing, behaviour and development.
- If any concerns, discuss with the parents whether the child is likely to have 'special educational needs' and arrange further action as appropriate.
- Measure height and plot on centile chart.
- Check for testicular descent unless previously fully descended at birth.

- If there are any concerns about the child's hearing, perform or arrange for, a hearing test.

Forty-eight to sixty-six months (school entry)

(These tests/assessments may be carried out at different times and by different medical personnel: school nurse/ audiometrician/school doctor/clinic doctor, etc.)

- Enquire about parental and, where appropriate, teacher, concerns.
- Review pre-school records.
- Carry out physical examination if specifically indicated.
- Ausculate the child's heart if examination has not been carried out since 6–8 week check.
- Measure height and plot on centile chart.
- Check vision using a Snellen chart.
- Check hearing using 'sweep' pure tone audiometry test.

School years

- Further visual acuity checks at ages eight, eleven, and fourteen.
- Test colour vision using Ishihara plates at age eleven.
- Repeat height test only if there is concern about growth.

(Adapted from Hall, D. *Health for all children: a screening programme for child health surveillance.* (Oxford University Press 1989).)

Note: the screening tests outlined in this book cover the child up to the school entry examination as these are the tests normally carried out by the general practitioner or health visitor.

The Snellen test for screening for problems with visual acuity in school aged children, and the test for colour vision screening are normally performed by the school nurse who is specifically trained in the methodology.

The 'sweep' test using pure tone audiometry to detect hearing problems in school aged children is normally carried out by someone specifically trained in the methodology.

Training in these tests are considered to be beyond the scope of this book.

5 Neonatal examinations

These, with the majority of children, will be carried out in hospital by a paediatrician or obstetrician before the child is discharged. However, the neonatal examination is an extremely important part of overall child health surveillance, as the majority of severe abnormalities are picked up at this time. Because this booklet is designed mainly for those working in child health surveillance in the community, we felt it would be useful to outline here the kind of examinations carried out in the neonatal period, as a background to the subsequent programme.

The examination is normally carried out within forty-eight hours of birth and again before discharge. It usually includes:

- Weight
- Head circumference
- Skin—for colour, birthmarks, etc.
- Head shape
- Fontanelles

- Ears
- Eye appearance, including red reflex
- Palate—hard and soft
- Heart—auscultation
- Pulses
- Respiratory system
- Abdomen
- Umbilicus
- Genitalia—including descent of testes in boys
- Limbs—for normal formation, tone, and movement
- Anus—normal appearance
- Hips—for congenital dislocation.

Blood-screening tests

- Phenylketonuria (approximate incidence 1:10 000 live-births)—blood normally taken by heelprick 6–10 days after birth.
- For congenital hypothyroidism (incidence 1:3500)—blood normally taken at same time as blood for phenylketonuria, 6–10 days after birth.

Some districts in England and Wales are also screening for galactosaemia, sickle-cell disease, and cystic fibrosis.

Those carrying out child health surveillance in the community need to check and make sure that the results of the NEONATAL EXAMINATION and BLOOD TESTS are available.

6 Screening for congenital dislocation of the hip

1. Introduction

Congenital dislocation of the hip (CDH) is a potentially crippling disorder associated with a high degree of handicap and orthopaedic problems in childhood and adulthood if not recognized early.

2. Incidence of CDH

The incidence of CDH in Caucasians is about two in every thousand live births. The incidence of hip instability is however, ten times as high as this; and although the majority spontaneously become normal, screening techniques cannot distinguish between those cases which will and those which will not resolve. Waiting for the natural evolution and postponing treatment is wasting time, and the outcome deteriorates. The earlier the diagnosis and treatment the better the outlook.

3. Aetiology and risk factors

Aetiology of CDH is still unclear.
  Risk factors associated with an increase of incidence:
  * genetic   —familial history of CDH
              —female
  * gestational—oligohydramnios
              —uterine malformations
              —first baby
              —fetal growth retardation

        —breech presentation
        —Caesarean section
- other congenital malformation (especially of the foot)

4. Screening tests

(a) Modified Ortolani–Barlow manoeuvre
The following conditions must be followed:

1. The infant must be undressed from the waist downwards.
2. The examiner's hands should be warm, the examination gentle, and the baby relaxed.
3. The infant lies on his/her back with legs towards the examiner, and the hips abducted and fully flexed.
4. For examination of the left hip the examiner steadies the infant's pelvis between the thumb of his left hand, on the symphysis pubis, and the fingers, under the sacrum.
5. The upper thigh of the left leg is grasped by the examiner's right hand, with the middle digit over the greater trochanter, with the flexed leg held in the palm, and with the thumb on the inner side of the thigh opposite the lesser trochanter.
6. An attempt is now made to move the femoral head in turn gently forwards into and backwards out of the acetabulum.
7. In the first part of the manoeuvre the middle digit is pressed upon the greater trochanter in an attempt to relocate the posteriorly displaced head of the femur forwards into the acetabulum. If the head is felt to move (usually not more than 0.5 cm), with or without a palpable and/or audible 'clunk', then dislocation is present.
8. The second part of the manoeuvre tests for instability. With the thumb on the inner side of the thigh, backward pressure is applied to the head of the femur. If the latter is

felt to move backwards over the labrum (the fibrocartilagi-neous rim of the acetabulum) on to the posterior aspect of the joint capsule (again a movement of not more than 0.5 cm, and often accompanied by a 'clunk') then the hip is said to be *subluxatable* or *unstable.*

9. To examine the right hip the role of the examiner's hand is reversed.

(b) Abduction test

This test should be carried out at all ages, as limitation of abduction is the most important sign of dislocation.

With the infant lying on his/her back and hips flexed to 90 degrees:

1. either both hips can be abducted at the same time—with limitation noted in one hip or the other, or both in bilateral dislocation (thighs normally abduct to 75°); or

2. one hip at a time can be abducted; but the pelvis must be stabilized with the other hand to prevent 'tipping'.

5. Classical signs

1. Limitation of hip abduction (persistent and less than 75°).

2. Shortening of the leg on the affected side and asymmetry between the two sides. (With hips flexed, compare knee levels. It is an above-knee shortening.)

3. Asymmetrical skin creases; check in supine and prone positions (not very reliable, but it can help the diagnosis).

4. Flattening of the buttock on the affected side in the prone position.

5. Leg posture: the affected side tends to be held in partial lateral rotation, flexion, and abduction.

6. Gait

The incidence of failure to walk by eighteen months of age in children with CDH is four times greater than in normal children. However, 80 per cent of children with CDH stand and walk at normal age. A child with unilateral dislocation may limp or fall to the affected side. If CDH is bilateral the gait is waddling. After two years the child cannot balance on the affected leg.

7. When to do the tests

Age	Tests			
	Ortolani–Barlow manoeuvre	Hip abduction	Classical signs	Gait
at birth	+	+	+	−
at discharge	+	+	+	−
6–8 weeks	+	+	+	−
6–9 months	−	+	+	−
15–21 months	−	+	+	+
walking	−	+	+	+

8. Action

Refer for orthopaedic opinion:

(a) all children with an abnormal response to the Ortolani–Barlow manoeuvre;

(b) all children with one or more 'classical signs';

(c) all children with gait problems;

(d) all children whose parents are worried about their child's gait; and

(e) any child for whom there are any doubts, when the child has one or more risk factors.

9. Follow-up

Always check the final outcome of children referred.

Further reading

Berman, L. and Klenerman, L. (1986). Ultrasound screening for hip abnormalities; preliminary findings in 1001 neonates. *British Medical Journal*, **293**, 719-22.

Department of Health and Social Security (1986). *Screening for the detection of congenital dislocation of the hip*. HMSO, London.

Dunn, P. M. (1987). Screening for congenital dislocation of the hip. In *Progress in child health* (ed. J. A. Macfarlane), Vol. 3. Churchill Livingstone, Edinburgh.

Dwyer, N. St. J. P. (1987). Congenital dislocation of the hip; to screen or not to screen? *Archives of Disease in Childhood*, **62**, 635-7.

Fixsen, J. (1985). Congenital dislocation of the hip. In *Progress in child health* (ed. J. A. Macfarlane), Vol. 2. Churchill Livingstone, Edinburgh.

Frankenburg, W. K. (1981). To screen or not to screen. Congenital dislocation of the hip. *American Journal of Public Health*, **71**, 1311-12.

Heikkila, E., Ryooppy, S., and Louhimo, I. (1984). Late diagnosis in congenital dislocation of the hip. *Acta Orthopaedica Scandinavica*, **55**, 256-60.

Knox, E. G., Armstrong, E. H., and Lancashire, R. J. (1987). Effectiveness of screening for congenital dislocation of the hip. *Journal of Epidemiology and Community Health*, **41**, 283-9.

Information booklet for parents—Lee, A. and Spinks, P. 'Hip displacement and your child'. West Berkshire Health Authority.

Training video 'Screening for congenital dislocation of the hip', bought or hired from Plymouth Medical Films, 33 New St. Barbican, Plymouth, PL1 2NA. Tel. (0752) 267711.

7 Screening for visual problems

1. Introduction

Although the most serious visual defects are usually apparent at the neonatal examination or subsequently become evident to the parents, screening for visual impairment is essential for the identification of the less serious but more common problems.

2. Prevalence of some visual defects in childhood (per 1000 live births)

- squint—30–40/1000
- hypermetropia—30/1000
- astigmatism—30/1000
- myopia—10 (6 years) to 200 (16 years)/1000
- cataract—0.2 (bilateral) + 0.2 (unilateral)/1000
- optic atrophy—0.2/1000
- retrolental fibroplasia—0.2/1000
- retinoblastoma—0.1/1000
- colour vision defects—80/1000 boys
                        — 4/1000 girls
- amblyopia—20 (in general population)/1000
- (disabling visual impairment is present in 2-4/10 000

3. Aetiologies and risk factors

Causes of severe visual handicap in children

- congenital conditions (inherited disorders of the eye or multiple malformative syndromes, prenatal infections, rubella, etc.)—70 per cent

- optic atrophy—10 per cent
- retrolental fibroplasia—6 per cent
- retinoblastoma—4 per cent
- other (postnatal eye or brain infection or trauma, perinatal insults)—10 per cent

Risk factors associated with an increase of visual problems

- familial history of—squints
                    —ocular disorders before six years
                    —wearing glasses before ten years
                    —retinoblastoma, glaucoma, etc.
- prenatal infection—rubella
- perinatal insults
- recognizable genetic syndromes and other malformations
- postnatal infections (eye or brain)
- trauma (head or eye)
- oxygen therapy in the neonatal period
- child abuse (head-shaking)

4. The tests

(a) History

- check risk factors (see above)
- does the mother think the child sees normally?
- Is the mother worried about the child's eyes?

(b) Ocular appearance

- Do the child's eyes look normal? Is the gaze steady?

(c) Ask about any parental concern

(d) Active questioning of parents:
Does the baby:
- look at the parents?
- follow moving objects with the eyes?
- fixate small objects?

5. **When to screen**

Age at test	(a) History	(b) Ocular appearance	(c) Parental concern	(d) Active questioning
Perinatal	+	+	+	−
6–8 weeks	+	+	+	+
7–9 months	−	+	+	+
$1\frac{1}{2}$–2 years	−	+	+	+
3–$3\frac{1}{2}$ years	−	+	+	+
$4\frac{1}{2}$–$5\frac{1}{2}$ years	−	+	+	+

6. **Action**

Refer:
- if there is any concern about the child's vision
- if risk factors are present

7. **Follow-up**

Always check out the final outcome of the children referred.

Further reading

Catford, J. *et al.* (1984). 'Squints—a sideways look'. In *Progress in child health*, vol. 1 (ed. J. A. Macfarlane), pp. 38–50. Churchill Livingstone, Edinburgh.

Egan, D. F. and Brown, R. (1984). Vision testing of young children in the age range 18 months to $4\frac{1}{2}$ years. *Child Care, Health and Development*, **10**, 381–90.

Hall, S. M., Pugh, A. G., and Hall, D. M. B. (1982). Vision screening in the under-5s. *British Medical Journal*, **285**, 1096–8.

Ingram, R. M., Holland, W. W., Walker, C., Wilson, J. M., Arnold, P. E., and Dally, S. (1986). Screening for visual defects in preschool children. *British Journal of Ophthalmology*, **70**, 16–21.

Kohler, L. (1984). Early detection and screening programmes for children in Sweden. In *Progress in Child Health* (ed. J. A. Macfarlane), Vol. 1. Churchill Livingstone, Edinburgh.

Stewart-Brown, S. (1987). Visual defects in school children: screening policy and educational implications. In *Progress in child health*, vol. 3 (ed. J. A. Macfarlane), pp. 14–37. Churchill Livingstone, Edinburgh.

Stewart-Brown, S. L., Haslum, M. N., and Howlett, B. (1988). Preschool vision screening; a service in need of rationalisation. *Archives of Disease in Childhood*, **63**, 356–9.

Taylor, D. and Rice, N. S. C. (1982). Congenital cataracts, a cause of preventable child blindness. *Archives of Disease in Childhood*, **57**, 165–6.

8   Screening for hearing problems

1. Introduction

All long-standing bilateral hearing impairments in children are significant because they may adversely affect the child's linguistic, educational, social, and emotional well-being by preventing the acquisition of normal language, and thus also obstructing normal social interaction.

Early diagnosis is therefore essential.

2. Prevalence of bilateral sensorineural hearing impairment in children:

- mild (35–50 dB)—13/1000 children;
- moderate (50–70 dB)—2/1000 children;
- severe (>70 dB)—1/1500 children.

(Twenty-five per cent of children under five years, and five to ten per cent of those over five years experience some transient conductive hearing-loss at some time.)

3. Aetiological factors

Children at increased risk of deafness

(These factors appear in 8 per cent of all children, and include 70–80 per cent of those with early deafness.)

- Family history of hereditary childhood deafness;
- rubella, 'flu', or other prenatal non-bacterial infections in first trimester of pregnancy;
- physical malformations, especially around the ear;
- prematurity;
- severe neonatal jaundice;
- drugs (aminoglycosides);
- meningitis, encephalitis, mumps, or measles;
- cerebral palsy;
- recurrent otitis media;
- head injury;
- birth asphyxia; and
- facial malformations, or Down's or Turner's syndrome.

4. Main causes of hearing-loss

(a) Conductive hearing-loss

Conductive hearing-loss is caused by mucous secretions ('glue') accumulating in the middle ear. This occurs as a result of blockage of the Eustachian tubes. These secretions interfere with the normal movements of the ossicles and ear-drum; the condition is called secretory otitis media (SOM).

Children with Down's syndrome, Turner's syndrome, facial malformations, or cleft palate, are at particular risk of developing a conductive hearing-loss.

● Note—*wax does not normally cause hearing-loss in children.*

(b) Sensorineural hearing-loss

This can be congenital or acquired. The inner ear (cochlea) or the nerve pathways are damaged. The hearing-loss is profound and permanent.

(c) Mixed conductive and sensorineural hearing-loss

5. Method of screening in the community

A screening programme for hearing problems needs age-appropriate validated tests to be well applied to whole populations of children. An improvement brought about after careful training in the carrying out of the distraction test, for example, has been known to increase the rate of detection of deaf children from 20 per cent to 70 per cent (McCormick 1988, p. 45-6).

(a) Utilization of parental suspicion

Parents' observations of their babies' reactions to sounds are very reliable indicators for the diagnosis of hearing problems—this can be aided by the parents' having a check-list to complete about their observations of their child's response to sounds (McCormick 1988).

- Ask parents if they have any concern about their child's hearing.
- Check for risk factors.
- Note if parents mention that the child:
  - —makes a limited number of sounds;
  - —screams in a high-pitched voice;
  - —has a funny voice;
  - —doesn't turn towards sounds;
  - —has an absence of the startle reflex between birth and four months; or
  - —shows the presence of the startle reflex between four months and one year.

(b) Distraction test

The aim of the test is to identify on clear 'pass/fail' criteria those babies who need further investigation.

Definition of 'pass/fail':

- —If there is any parental concern—present each sound at least twice.
- —Pass: A definite and full head-turn in the direction of the sound.

If there is a good response to the first presentation of the sound—and no parental concern—pass.

- —Fail: A failure to orientate to any of the sounds on either side.

If the baby fails to respond to the first presentation of any sound, present twice more (not consecutively). The baby should respond to two out of three presentations of each sound. If he/she fails to respond to any sound presented twice,—re-test in one month.

To optimize the performance of the test these conditions must be followed:

- The test should be conducted in the quietest available surroundings, whether in clinic or home—maximum ambient noise=35/40 dB.

- Two trained personnel are needed (the 'tester' and the 'distractor'), both of whom need to have normal hearing.

- *The tester's role is:* to present the stimulus at the appropriate time; the distractor decides if the baby passes or fails.

- *The distractor's role is:* to attract and hold the baby's attention briefly. This is preferably done with finger-play; but a suitable toy may be used for a restless child. Movement is then stopped, or the toy covered, releasing the baby's attention. This is the ideal moment for presentation of the sound-stimulus by the tester. The distractor controls the test and decides if the baby passes or fails.

- Stimuli of known frequency characterization must be used. It is essential to use both high- and low-frequency stimuli at minimal levels (35 dB measured at the test ear).

- Sound-signals should be presented at ear-level, at a standard distance of 3 feet (1 metre) from the test ear, at an angle of 45° from the child's head behind the child's peripheral visual field (note that visual stimuli are more dominant than auditory, and that the sphere of visual attention is wider (3 metres) than that of auditory attention (1 metre). *Always* keep the sound source behind the mother's chair-back (see diagram, Fig. 8.1).

The order of testing is:

(a) Test for normal head movements by getting the baby to follow an object visually.

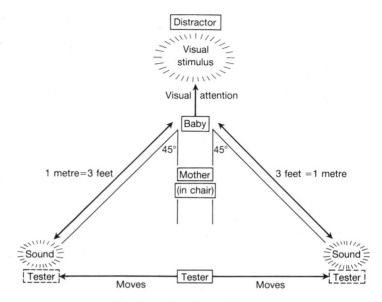

Fig. 8.1. The distraction test.

(b) Then test using sounds on left and right, each sound being presented twice, for approximately 3–five seconds, on each side.

Order of sounds:

1. Minimal voiced sentence, for example, 'Hello, baby, how are you?', but with no 'ss' sounds.

2. Low, quiet, voiced 'oo-oo' or 'mm-mm'.

3. The sound 'ss', 'ss' (as in 'face').

4. High-tone Manchester rattle agitated gently.

(c) Test for visual responses and other false responses by presenting 'no-sound' trials, using the rattle and movement of the tester—but *no* sound.

The only acceptable response is a turn of the head to the source of the sound. Other responses—for example, a stilling of activity, a change of expression, or eye-movements—are not acceptable in screening tests. After the baby has turned show him/her the sound source. The baby should respond correctly to the four sounds on each side (see pass/fail criteria p. 29).

Pitfalls

Extreme care must be taken to avoid:

—auditory clues (footsteps, rustling of clothes or carpets, creaking floors);

—visual clues (shadows, moving into the child's peripheral visual field, reflections in mirrors or in one-way observation screens—it may be necessary to switch off certain lights or to draw curtains);

—olfactory clues (for example, perfumes); and

—misinterpretation of random turning movements by the baby.

N.B. Regular checks using a sound-level meter should be carried out at six-monthly intervals, and testers and distractors should have their hearing tested every two years.

Speech discrimination test

This test is usually carried out on children aged three years or more. It is not used as a 'screening' test—but is useful when there is suspicion of hearing-loss in children of this age.

Seven toys, or pictures, are used. Present the toys, or pictures, to the child, naming them clearly. Place them in front of the child and ask the child to point to each toy to ensure the vocabulary is understood. The examiner should then move (in stages, if necessary to hold the child's attention) to 6–10 feet (2–3 metres) from the child and to the (right) or (left) side, and then, without showing the mouth, to avoid lip-reading, should ask the child to 'show me the . . .', naming each toy in turn. The beginning of the sentence should always be said at normal voice-level, and then the name of the toy at reduced voice-level (40 dB).

Suitable toys to use are:
—ball
—doll
—plane
—car
—stick
—brick
—ship.

These single-syllable sounds cover low, middle, and high frequencies. Particular care is needed to check the level of voice—it must be *minimal* voice.

To pass the test the minimum response from the child should be to identify correctly four out of the five toys requested.

6. When to screen

Age of screening	Screening test
Ongoing throughout the first year	Parental checklist and direct parental questioning
7–9 months	Distraction test
5–6 years	School audiogram

Note: at 7–9 months do NOT allow for prematurity; test at birth-date age.

Children should have a hearing test *any* time that the parents or anyone else is concerned as to whether the child can hear or not.

7. Action

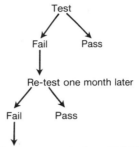

Fig. 8.2. The action sequence when screening for hearing problems.

When to refer:

1. Refer immediately to ENT via the GP if the baby/child appears to be profoundly, bilaterally deaf.
2. Do *not* omit standard referral procedure if the baby/child has a cold during the two tests.
3. If a baby/child fails the hearing test on the re-test the eardrums should be examined and appropriately treated. If the baby/child has bilateral serous otitis a referral to ENT or to Audiology may be indicated.
4. Direct referrals from health visitors can be made to hearing therapists in ENT with GP consent. Keep a note of your local therapist and of further referral possibilities, perhaps in the following form:

   Your local Hearing Therapist is...
   Tel..
   For children who are difficult to test contact..............................
   Tel......................................

   All field-staff should attend regular updating sessions, and have their own hearing tested every two years.

References and further reading

Black, N. A. (1985). Surgery for glue ear—the determinants of an epidemic. In *Progress in Child Health* (ed. J. A. Macfarlane), Vol. 2. Churchill Livingstone, Edinburgh.

Boothman, R. and Orr, N. (1978). Screening for deafness in the first year of life. *Archives of Disease in Childhood*, **53**, 570-3.

Department of Health and Social Security (1981). *The ACSHIP Report* (Chairman J. C. Balantyne). Advisory committee on services for hearing impaired people. Report of the sub-committee for hearing impaired children. DHSS.

Grant, H. R., Quiney, R. E., Mercer, D. M., and Lodge, S. (1988). Cleft palate and glue ear. *Archives of Disease in Childhood*, **63**, 176-9.

Hall, D. M. B. and Hill, P. (1986). When does secretory otitis media affect language development? *Archives of Disease in Childhood*, **61**, 42-7.

Hitchings, V. and Haggard, M. P. (1983). Incorporation of parental suspicions in screening infants. *British Journal of Audiology*, **17**, 71-5.

Martin, J. A. M. and Moore, W. J. (1979). *Childhood deafness in the European community.* Commission of the European Communities, HMSO (EUR 6413), London.

McCormick, B. (1977). The toy discrimination test: an aid for screening the hearing of children above a mental age of two years. *Public Health*, **91**, 67-9.

McCormick, B. (1983). Hearing screening by health visitors; a critical appraisal of the distraction test. *Health Visitor*, **56**, 449-51.

McCormick, B. (1988). *Screening for hearing impairment in young children.* Croom Helm, London.

Newton, V. E. (1985). Aetiology of bilateral sensori-neural hearing loss in young children. *Journal of Laryngology and Otology* Supplement 10.

Paradise, J. L. (1981). Otitis media during early life; how hazardous to development? A critical review of the evidence. *Pediatrics*, **68**, 869-73.

Sade, J. (1979). *Secretory otitis media and its sequelae.* Monographs in Clinical Otolaryngology, No. 1. Churchill Livingstone, Edinburgh.

Yeates, S. (1981). *Development of hearing.* MTP Press, Lancaster.

Video: 'Screening and Surveillance for Hearing Impairment in Young Children', Nottingham Health Authority. Obtainable from: Audio Visual Educational Services, Queens Medical Centre, Nottingham.

9 Screening for heart disease

1. Introduction

It is important that doctors involved in surveillance can distinguish between innocent and pathological murmurs, and are able to identify the other signs and symptoms of congenital heart disease (CHD).

2. Incidence

Six to eight children in a thousand are born with congenital heart disease. However, an 'innocent' or 'physiological' murmur is present in more than 50 per cent of all children and adolescents.

3. Aetiology and risk factors

The aetiologies of congenital heart diseases are numerous, and usually unknown; but some risk factors that are associated with a higher incidence of CHD are:

(a) family history of CHD or other malformations (i.e. renal);

(b) pregnancy problems (infections, X-ray, alcohol, tobacco, drugs, drug abuse, systemic diseases, etc.);

(c) birth problems (low or high birthweight, anoxia, resuscitation);

(d) neonatal problems (infection, respiratory); and

(e) recognizable genetic syndromes or other malformations.

4. Age at examination

At birth, at from six to eight weeks, and opportunistically up to four and a half to five and a half years, at which age examination should be carried out on school entry.

5. Symptoms which should alert the examiner

1. Shortness of breath on exertion.
2. Chest pains.
3. Excessive tiredness.
4. Palpitations or syncope.
5. Feeding problems and/or failure to thrive.
6. Late walking.
7. Excessive sweating.
8. Squatting.
9. Recurrent low-respiratory-tract infections.

6. Examination

(a) The murmur

A murmur should be listened to:

1. Standing or sitting and supine.
2. In inspiration and expiration.
3. Over the left and right of the front chest, the back, and the neck.

4. If a murmur is continuous and is transmitted to the neck, listen with the child supine with his/her legs higher than his/her head. If the murmur is a venous hum the diastolic component will disappear.

Innocent murmurs are commonly:
1. Systolic with no diastolic component (except venous hum).
2. Soft, graded $\frac{3}{6}$ or less.
3. Short ejection murmurs.
4. Well localized without radiation.
5. Never accompanied by a thrill.
6. Louder with exercise, fever, or anxiety.
7. Accompanied by no other signs and/or symptoms of cardiac disease.
8. Not accompanied by other abnormal cardiac sounds.

Pathological murmurs (those calling for referral)
1. All diastolic murmurs.
2. All pansystolic murmurs.
3. All late systolic murmurs.
4. Louder than $\frac{3}{6}$ grade and/or accompanied by a thrill.
5. Continuous murmurs (except venous hum).
6. Any murmur heard at the back.
7. Most murmurs transmitted to the neck (except venous hums).
8. Mumurs associated with signs or/and symptoms of cardiac disease.

(b) Other signs of cardiac disease
Consider:
1. Heart sounds—especially loudness and wide or fixed splitting of second sound, or clicks.
2. Central cyanosis.
3. Rapid respiratory rate.
4. Abnormal apex beat or precordium bulge.

5. Clubbing.
6. Peripheral arterial pulses (radial/brachial and femoral).
7. Blood-pressure if appropriate cuff is available (that is, one covering $\frac{2}{3}$ of upper arm with balloon encircling arm).

7. Action

Refer to specialized clinic if:

1. There are suspicions or *doubts* as to whether the murmur is pathological.
2. The child has symptoms and/or signs of heart disease.
3. The parents are anxious after discussion.

Notify health visitor of referral.

If you consider the murmur innocent continue the routine surveillance programme. Explain to the parents that the child can lead a normal life, and do NOT prescribe antibiotic prophylaxis. Note on records the presence of any murmur, and the discussion with the parents.

8. Follow-ups

Always check up on the final outcome of children who are referred.

Further reading

McLaren, M. J., Lachman, A. S., Pocock, W. A., and Barlow, J. B. (1980). Innocent murmurs and third heart sounds in Black schoolchildren. *British Heart Journal*, **43**, 67–73.

Newburger, J. W., Rosenthal, A., Williams, R. G., Fellows, K., and Miettinen, O. S. Invasive tests in the initial evaluation of heart murmurs in children. *New England Journal of Medicine*, **308**, 61–4.

Raftery, E. B. and Holland, W. W. (1966). Examination of the heart: an investigation into variation. *American Journal of Epidemiology*, **85**, 438–44.

Rosenthal, A. (1984). How to distinguish between innocent and pathologic murmurs in childhood. *Pediatric Clinics of North America*, **31**, 1229–40.

Scott, D. J., Rigby, M. L., Miller, G. A. H., and Shinebourne, E. A. (1984). The presentation of symptomatic heart disease in infancy based on 10 years' experience (1973–82). Implications for the provision of services. *British Heart Journal*, **52**, 248–57.

10 Screening for abnormalities of head circumference

1. Introduction

Head-circumference measurement may have an important diagnostic significance in the first few years of life, and is particularly valuable in infants up to one year of age. The routine examination of babies in child-health clinics, in hospital, or at home should include the measurement of the maximum circumference of the skull, and plotting this on a percentile chart, the reason being that the size of the skull depends in large part on the growth of the cranial contents. By definition 3 per cent of babies will have heads <3rd centile and 3 per cent > than the 97th centile.

2. Aetiologies

The commonest causes of a small head are as follows:

   —small baby

  —familial feature
  —mental subnormality (including congenital diseases)
  —craniosynostosis
  —abnormal neurological development
but no precise prevalence rates of these causes are available.

The commonest causes for an unusually large head are:
  —large baby
  —familial feature
  —hydrocephalus
  —hydranencephaly
  —megalencephaly
  —subdural effusion
  —cerebral tumour
  —craniosynostosis
  —mucopolysaccharidosis

No precise prevalence rates of these causes are available, but, in a Sheffield study, out of 557 children referred because of a large head-size, and almost always otherwise well, 384 had increased intracranial pressure, 140 were normal, mostly with a large head as a familial feature, and 33 had other abnormalities (Lorber 1981).

Some of these conditions, notably the subdural effusion, hydrocephalus, cerebral tumour, and craniosynostosis, can benefit from an early diagnosis and subsequent treatment. In some other cases a rapid diagnosis can allow genetic counselling.

3. The test

Accuracy is important in the measurement of head circumference. Inaccuracies in technique may result in significant errors when plotting the value on the centile chart. No matter who performs the measurement, they must be aware of the importance of accurate technique.

The head circumference can be measured with a paper or plastic tape, as the maximum circumference around the supraorbital ridges and glabella (anteriorly), and that part of the occiput that gives the maximal circumference (posteriorly). The tape must be pulled tight to compress the hair; and the measurement is read to the nearest millimetre. If the head is abnormally shaped, the serial measurements may best be made by positioning the tape over the points of the forehead and occiput that give the maximal circumference. Cloth, linen, or plastic tapes may stretch with age, and need to be periodically checked against wooden or steel standards. Thick tapes will slide about as well. The head-circumference measurement should ideally be taken three times at the same session, averaged, and then plotted on a centile chart.

4. When to measure

Before discharge from hospital, and then at six to eight weeks of age.

The measurement should be written in figures as well as plotted on a centile chart. If the two measurements are following the same centile line, and if there is no concern at six to eight weeks, no further measurement is needed. If there is any concern about a baby's growth, health, or development, the baby's head circumference should always be measured and recorded.

5. Action

In the face of an abnormal value the obvious potential source of error must be checked before any deductions can be made, namely: is the method of measurement correct? (In a

nine-month-old child an error of 2 cm in the head circumference changes centile ranking from 50 to 95.) Was the age
correctly assessed? For example, $4\frac{1}{2}$ months is not 5 months!
Has the gestational age been considered? Action in the case
of a large head which is increasing in size is much more
urgent than with a small head.

So if the head circumference, after accurate measurement,
is:

(a) Above the 97th centile.
(b) Below the 3rd centile.
(c) Crossing percentiles.
(d) In great disparity with the weight centile.

Then:

1. Discuss with the parents.
2. Ask the parents about symptoms, developmental problems, and obstetric or perinatal problems.
3. Check familial history of large/small head-size.
4. Measure the parents' head circumference.
5. Have the child checked by the clinic doctor.
6. If no other signs or symptoms—measure again in one
   month.
7. If after one month the head circumference is not growing
   away from centile lines, treat as normal. If growing away
   from centiles: refer—with centile chart.

When to refer:
1. Child with symptoms.
2. Child with developmental problems.
3. Head circumference curve that deviates away from the
   97th centile or the 3rd centile or crosses centile ranks
   without the same evolution of the weight curve.
4. Parental anxiety.
5. When you suspect something is wrong although you cannot tell exactly what.

6. Follow-up

It is essential to check up on the final outcome of a child who is referred.

References and further reading

Day, R. E. and Schutt, W. H. (1979). Normal children with large heads; benign familial megalencephaly. *Archives of Disease in Childhood*, **54**, 512–17.

Dennis, M., Fitz, C. R., Oxtley, C. T., Sugar, J., Harwood-Nash, D. C., Hendrick, E. B., Hoffman, J. J., and Humphreys, R. P. (1981). The intelligence of hydrocephalic children. *Archives of Neurology*, **38**, 607–15.

Lorber, J. and Priestley, B. L. (1981). Children with large heads. *Developmental Medicine and Child Neurology*, **23**, 494–504.

11 Screening for weight problems

1. Introduction

It can be argued that 'weight' by itself is not a screening test (Hall 1989), as it does not fulfil the criteria of 'screening' tests. However routine weighing is carried out, particularly in child-health clinics, and so weight is included here for the sake of completeness. Weight-gain is the most widely used clinical measurement of growth in post-natal life, being an index of not only illness and poor nutrition but also in some cases of emotional deprivation. Weight should be routinely measured in child-health clinics or at home, and the results plotted on a centile chart so that early diagnosis and intervention can take place.

2. Aetiologies and prevalences of poor growth

- Underfeeding (the commonest cause).
- Environmental and socio-psychological deprivation.
- Coeliac disease, cystic fibrosis, other malabsorptions.
- Other chronic organic diseases and chronic infections.
- Recognizable congenital syndromes.
- Neuroendocrine or metabolic diseases.

Exact prevalence rates are not available.

Measurement

It must be remembered that there may be considerable apparent variation of the weight of babies on a day-to-day basis, as a result of:

(a) Whether the baby's bladder is full or empty.
(b) How recently the baby has been fed.
(c) The use of different scales.
(d) The baby not always being weighed unclothed.
(e) If weighed clothed, the amount of clothing worn (seasonal differences).

All these factors need to be taken into account.

3. The test

Accurate measurement of weight is required, so certain conditions must be followed:

1. The scale must be in order (calibrated).
2. The baby should be naked (whenever possible).

3. After six months of age weight is measured to the last complete 0.1 kg.
4. If the child is restless it may become necessary to weigh him/her held by the mother, and then subtract the mother's weight.
5. All measurements should be entered on a suitable growth chart.
6. Corrections should be made for gestational age.
7. Measurements should be dated and recorded in figures, as well as plotted on the centile chart.

4. When to weigh

Accurate measurements of weight should be made up to two years of age, whenever the child attends clinic. In the normal child too frequent weighing is, as a rule, undesirable, because it is likely to produce anxiety and unnecessarily worry parents, and because minor diseases may temporarily slow the weight progress without any special significance. Obviously where there is concern about a child's weight increased frequency is appropriate.

5. Action

If the child's weight is below the 3rd centile or is crossing percentile lines downwards over several weeks, certain things must be checked:

- how accurate was the technique used?
- what was the birthweight and how did it correlate with gestational age?
- are all the family small?
- when did the slowing of the weight-gain rate take place?
- is the child being adequately fed?

- ask parents about symptoms (gastrointestinal, developmental and other).
- have the child checked by the clinic doctor.
- discuss the matter with parents.

When to refer:
1. Children below the 3rd centile.
2. Children who consistently cross centile lines downwards.
3. When you suspect something is wrong although you cannot tell exactly what.

6. Follow-up

It is essential to check up on the final outcome of the child you refer.

N.B.: It is very difficult to draw a line between what is 'good' and what is 'excessive' nutrition. A child may be overweight owing to excess of fat tissue (true obesity), to a heavier skeletal frame, or to a greater amount of muscular tissue. The commonest causes of obesity are familial idiopathic and excessive intake of food, which may not be associated with lack of activity. Some organic diseases (neuro-endocrine and congenital) can present with overweight. Note especially the fat and small child in this context. However, although obesity in adulthood has been associated with an increase of morbidity and mortality, there is still a lack of evidence that supports the need for or the feasibility of screening. Nonetheless, a child with gross obesity—when recognized—should be referred for a medical consultation.

Further reading

Dowdney, L., Skuse, D., Heptinstall, E., Puckering, C., and Zur-Szpiro, S. (1987). Growth retardation and developmental delay amongst inner-city children. *Journal of Child Psychology and Psychiatry,* **28**, 529–41.

Evans, T. J. and Davies, D. P. (1977). Failure to thrive at the breast. *Archives of Disease in Childhood,* **52**, 974–5.

Goldson, E. (1987). Failure to thrive; an old problem re-visited. In *Progress in child health* (ed. J. A. Macfarlane), Vol. 3. Churchill Livingstone, Edinburgh.

Hall, D. (1989). *Health for all children. A programme for child health surveillance.* Oxford University Press.

Heptinstall, E., Puckering, C., Skuse, D., Dowdney, L., and Zur-Szpiro, S. (1987). Nutrition and meal-time behaviour in families of growth-retarded children. *Human Nutrition: Applied Nutrition*, **41**, 390–402.

Mitchell, W. G., Gorrell, R. W., and Greenberg, R. A. (1980). Failure to thrive; a study in a primary care setting; epidemiology and follow-up. *Pediatrics*, **65**, 971–7.

12 Screening for height problems

1. Introduction

Measurement of height is an important clinical assessment of skeletal growth, and should be performed from two years of age onwards. Results should always be plotted on a percentile chart.

2. Aetiologies of short stature

–Familial
–Psychosocial
–Low birthweight

—Endocrine disorders (growth-hormone deficiency, hypothyroidism, etc.; hypothalamus-pituitary-glandular axis
disorders)
—Organic diseases—coeliac disease, cystic fibrosis, and
other chronic conditions, or malabsorptions
—Congenital syndromes (Turner and other)

(In the Oxfordshire study of 227 children referred for short
stature, 60 per cent were 'short normal', 9 per cent hypothyroidism, 7 per cent had Turner syndrome, 6 per cent had
growth hormone deficiency and 18 per cent manifested other
causes (Aynsley Green 1983).)

3. The test

Two recommended measuring instruments are (1) the
'Oxford Growth Screening Wall Chart' and (2) The Micro-
toise. Accuracy of measurement depends on the following
conditions:

1. Children must be measured with bare feet (no shoes or
   socks), with the back of the heels against the wall and the
   bottom of the heels on the floor, and the feet together.
2. The head must face forward.
3. The back edge of the eye should be at the same level as
   the external auditory canal.
4. The centre of the back of the head should be against the
   chart/wall.
5. Take the height from the top of the head.

4. When to measure

Routinely at two to three years and four and a half to five and
a half years. More frequently if there is a problem.

5. Action

A study done in Scotland revealed that although 70 per cent of mothers whose children's heights fell below the 3rd centile recognized that the child had a short stature, only 10 per cent sought advice. This outlines the need for early screening and identification of such children in the community, to allow further investigation and treatment, since many of these causes can be treated and genetic counselling can also be undertaken where appropriate.

If there is concern on the part of health visitors or parents:

—Check the accuracy of techniques.
—Discuss the matter with parents.
—Check familial features of short stature by measuring and recording the parents' height.
—Check birth-size and birth weight.
—Ask parents about symptoms and developmental problems.
—Plot the height on a centile chart with previous heights, if possible.

When to consider for possible referral:
1. Children below the 3rd centile.
2. When parents and/or a health visitor think the child hasn't grown at all in the last year.
3. When you suspect something is wrong, although you cannot tell exactly what.

6. Follow-up

Always check up on the final outcome of children that you refer.

Note on the measurement of length in infants
● It has not yet been proved that the measurement of length

is sufficiently reliable to provide a good tool for screening purposes. However, if for any reason you have to measure length (that is, if parents ask you to, or where parents are convinced that although weight-gain is satisfactory the child is not growing in length), follow these instructions: measure the child lying down, with the lower orbital borders in the same vertical plane as the external auditory canal, knees flat, ankles gently pulled to stretch the infant, and feet held vertically. Two observers are needed. Two books are held, one against the top of the head and one against the soles of the feet. The distance between them is measured.

Note on tall children
- Tall children do not generally have organic disease, although they may have some orthopaedic problems. Psychological problems are, however, more important (especially in girls). Some congenital disorders (Soto's, Beckwith's, Marfan's, or Klinefelter's syndromes) may become evident through excessively tall stature. Tall children who come from short families may need investigation. However, for screening purposes, tallness lacks interest. Treatment of tall children is under review.

References and further reading

Aynsley Green, A. and Macfarlane, J. A. (1983). Method for the earlier recognition of abnormal stature. *Archives of Disease in Childhood*, **58**, 535-7.

Brook, C. D. G. (1982). *Growth assessment in childhood and adolescence.* Blackwell, Oxford.

Buchanan, C. R., Law, C. M., and Milner, R. D. G. (1987). Growth hormone in short, slowly growing children and those with Turner's syndrome. *Archives of Disease in Childhood*, **62**, 912-16.

Law, C. M. (1987). The disability of short stature. *Archives of Disease in Childhood*, **62**, 855-9.

Lyon, A. J., Preece, M. A., and Grant, D. B. (1985). Growth curve for girls with Turner syndrome. *Archives of Disease in Childhood*, **60**, 932–5.

Tanner, J. M. (1978). *Foetus into man.* Open Books, Wells.

Video: 'Screening for growth problems', available from: Plymouth Medical Films, 33, New Street, Barbican, Plymouth, PL1 2NA. Tel: (0752) 267711.

Contact for parents

Child Growth Foundation, 2, Mayfield Avenue, Chiswick, London W4 1PW. Tel: 01 995 0257.

13 Screening for cryptorchidism (undescended testis)

1. Introduction

Cryptorchidism is a condition in which one or both testes fail to descend to a normal position well down in the scrotum. It is one of the most common congenital abnormalities in males. The condition is bilateral in about 10 per cent of cases and in the majority of boys it occurs without any association with other malformations.

The incidence of undescended testis varies according to both the gestational age and the age of the child.

Table 13.1.

Age of child	Prevalence (%)
At birth	7.1*
2–3 months	1.6*
12 months	1.3

An additional 1.3 per cent develop UDT.
*The prevalence is considerably higher for low-birthweight babies.
Figures taken from the first twelve months of the Oxford Cryptorchidism Study Group (John Radcliffe Hospital Crytorchidism Study Group 1986a).

Most testes of boys who have cryptorchidism at birth descend spontaneously within the first year of life. *Those testes that are not well down in the scrotum at birth, or testes well down but associated with hydroceles, must be re-checked throughout the whole of the first five years of life.*

2. Aetiology and risk factors

The aetiology of cryptorchidism is still unclear, although hormonal causes seem to be implicated.

The accepted factors relating to an increase of incidence are:

- low birthweight—less than 2500 g;
- short gestation;
- associated clinical inguinal hernia.

Additional factors found in some studies:

- born to primigravidas;

- born to mothers aged less than twenty years;
- breech delivery; and
- mothers exposed to exogenous oestrogen therapy during the first trimester.

3. The reasons for identifying UDT

The reasons for screening for undescended testes are:

(a) Rising infertility rates (low sperm-counts occur in 100 per cent of bilateral untreated cases and 75 per cent of bilateral treated. The fertility-outcome advantage of therapy in unilateral cases is not clear).

(b) Increase in the cancer risk (undescended testes have a risk of developing cancer which is five times greater than that of the average population, although the advantages of an early intervention are still discussed).

(c) Increase in the risk of testicular torsion (which has a prevalence of 2 per cent in cases of undescended testis).

(d) Increase in the incidence of psychological problems ('castration complex').

(e) Cosmetic reasons.

(f) Correction of inguinal hernia (if associated).

(g) The operation can be performed at around one year.

(h) Diagnosis of the 3 per cent of cases in which one or both testes are absent, and of the 1 per cent of cases of ectopic testis.

4. The test

The screening test is to seek for a location of the testis well down in the scrotal sac.

Classification
1. Impalpable—abnormal, follow up.
2. High, or comes down and goes up again—abnormal, follow up.
3. Well down, or comes down and stays down—normal, no further examination needed.

The screening should be first carried out at birth, when the scrotum is relatively large, minimal subcutaneous fat exists, and the cremasteric reflex is absent. Palpation requires a warm and relaxed baby who is lying down, and a gentle examiner with warm hands. Each side of the scrotum should be examined separately.

If the testis is well down in the scrotal sac, then that testis can be passed as normal and does not need further examination.

If the testis cannot be felt in the scrotal sac then an attempt should be made to milk the testis down towards the scrotum with one hand, stroking along the line of the inguinal canal from the internal to the external ring, where it can be caught by the fingers of the other hand and pulled gently as far into the scrotum as it will come.

If the testis comes down and stays well down in the scrotum without any signs of retracting up again, then the test is normal and no further examination is needed.

If the testis is impalpable, high up, or comes down but shows *any* sign of retracting up again—follow up at six to eight weeks (see p. 51).

The retractile testis: In some boys, aged six months or more, the testis may retract out of the scrotum because of the cremasteric reflex. (The cremaster muscle retracts the testis when the skin is stroked on the front inner side of the thigh.) The cremasteric reflex is absent before the age of six months, but is most active between the second and seventh years of age, and may falsely increase the prevalence of apparent cryptorchidism during childhood.

5. **When to do the test**

At birth—for the whole population of boys (record results so that they are available in records available for the primary health-care team).

Thereafter—see flow diagram below.

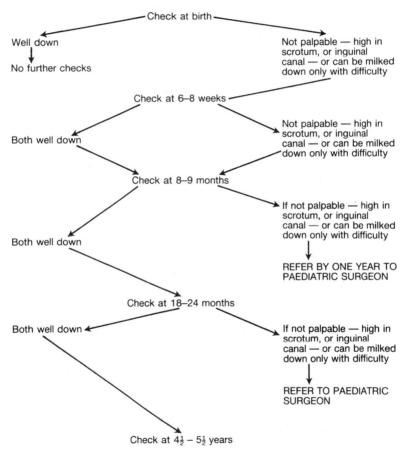

Fig. 13.1. Flow diagram of the sequence of screening tests for cryptorchidism over time.

6. Action

1. Boys whose testes are both well down at birth do *not* need to be followed.

2. Boys whose testes are *other* than well down in the scrotum at *birth*, unilaterally or bilaterally—that is, impalpable; or very high in the inguinal pouch or scrotum; or that are high, can be milked down, but retract up again: *Follow all of these until five years of age, because some that are in this group and then come down, may subsequently retract up again.*

3. *All boys whose testis/es have not completely descended by one year should be referred to a paediatric surgeon.*

4. Boys whose parents are anxious about their son's testes and/or want a further opinion—*refer.*

5. In case of doubt it is preferable to refer.

7. Follow-up

Always check the final outcome of those referred.

References and further reading

Atwell, J. D. (1985). Ascent of the testis: fact or fiction? *British Journal of Urology,* **57,** 474-7.

Chilvers, C., Dudley, N. E., Gough, M. H., Jackson, M. B., and Pike, M. C. (1986). Undescended testis: the effect of treatment on subsequent risk of subfertility and malignancy. *Journal of Pediatric Surgery,* **21,** 691-6.

Depue, R. H. (1984). Maternal and gestational factors affecting the risk of cryptorchidism and inguinal hernia. *International Journal of Epidemiology,* **13,** 311-18.

John Radcliffe Hospital Cryptorchidism Study Group (1986a). Cryptorchidism: an apparent substantial increase since 1960. *British Medical Journal,* **293,** 1404-6.

John Radcliffe Hospital Cryptorchidism Study Group (1986*b*). Boys with late descending testes: the source of cases of 'retractile testes' undergoing orchidopexy? *British Medical Journal*, **293**, 789–90.

John Radcliffe Hospital Cryptorchidism Study Group (1988). Clinical diagnosis of cryptorchidism. *Archives of Disease in Childhood*, **63**, 587–91.

Scorer, C. G. and Farrington, G. H. (1971). *Congenital deformities of the testis and epididymis.* Butterworth, London.

Index